Fatma Khalsi

VITAMIN D STATUS INASTHMATIC CHILDREN

Fatma Khalsi

VITAMIN D STATUS INASTHMATIC CHILDREN

ScienciaScripts

Imprint

Cover image: www.ingimage.com

This book is a translation from the original published under ISBN 978-620-6-71386-9.

Publisher:
Sciencia Scripts
is a trademark of
Dodo Books Indian Ocean Ltd. and OmniScriptum S.R.L publishing group

120 High Road, East Finchley, London, N2 9ED, United Kingdom
Str. Armeneasca 28/1, office 1, Chisinau MD-2012, Republic of Moldova, Europe
Printed at: see last page
ISBN: 978-620-7-67325-4

VITAMIN D STATUS IN ASTHMATIC CHILDREN

Introduction

Asthma in children is the most common respiratory disease worldwide. It is a major cause of morbidity and mortality [1]. Accurate assessment of its prevalence has been hampered by the heterogeneity of asthma definitions [1,2]. In a large French study conducted in 2016, this prevalence was estimated at 11% [2].

Asthma is a chronic inflammatory disorder of the airways, characterised by episodic or persistent symptoms such as dyspnoea, chest tightness, wheezing, mucus production and coughing. It is associated with variable obstruction of the airways, which are hyper-reactive to endogenous or exogenous stimuli. [1,3] These symptoms vary in time and intensity and are accompanied by a variable reduction in airflow [1]. This respiratory disorder is the result of a complex interaction between several genetic and environmental factors [3]. Among the environmental factors implicated in the pathogenesis of asthma, vitamin D status has attracted increasing interest over the last two decades [4]. In addition to its classic effects on bone, it has been described that vitamin D has an immunomodulatory effect via its receptor (VDR) and 1-alpha-hydroxylase, which are present in T and B lymphocytes, macrophages and antigen-presenting cells. For example, 25 hydroxy vitamin D (25 OH D) reduces the proliferation of T lymphocytes (in particular Thelper-1 [Th1] and Th17 lymphocytes) and the production of certain "proinflammatory" cytokines (in particular Il-2, Il-6 and IFN-y). It has also been described that the vitamin reduces respiratory infections, mainly viral, and improves lung function [4-6].

Over the last two decades, and since the increase in demand for methods of measuring monohydroxylated derivatives of vitamin D and the determination of reference values for vitamin D status, it has been shown that hypovitaminosis D is a widespread problem throughout the world, even in countries with a lot of sunshine [6-8]. Hypovitaminosis D is also widespread in children, particularly those suffering from asthma, and interferes with the control and severity of this condition [7-9].

The interaction between asthma and vitamin D has been extensively studied over the last two decades. This interaction takes place at several levels and has potential clinical implications for asthma patients, affecting the severity, control and prognosis of the disease.

Definitions :

Atopy: genetic predisposition to produce specific IgE antibodies to a given allergen

Sensitisation: positive results from allergological tests, such as skin tests or the measurement of specific IgE antibodies in blood samples.

Allergy: clinical manifestation linked to the development of an antigen-antibody reaction.

Allergy is therefore the clinical expression of sensitisation.

Asthma: a heterogeneous disorder characterised by chronic inflammation of the airways, manifested by symptoms such as wheezing, breathlessness, chest tightness and cough, which vary in time and intensity and are associated with variable limitation of expiratory flow [1].

I. General information on vitamin D :

Vitamin D is a fat-soluble vitamin with a dual origin:

- **Exogenous:** Dietary intake considered too low given the low content of foods consumed by most of the population; few people consume foods rich in vitamin D such as cod liver oil and wild salmon.
- **Endogenous,** resulting from skin neosynthesis under the effect of ultraviolet rays; long considered to be able to cover 70 to 90% of this vitamin's requirements [12].

The term "vitamin D" refers to vitamin D2, known as ergocalciferol, and vitamin D3, known as cholecalciferol, or one of its metabolites.

25-hydroxyvitamin D (25 OH D) is the storage form of vitamin D and is the marker of an individual's vitamin D status. [7,10]

The biological parameter that defines vitamin D status is the serum concentration of 25-OH vitamin D3 [25OHD3]. Although 1,25 (OH) 2 D3 is the active metabolite of vitamin D (500 times more active), it is not a representative marker of vitamin D status [7].

Determining reference values for vitamin D status :

It is impossible to determine reference values for vitamin D status using the gausse curve because of the many factors that influence vitamin D levels (skin pigmentation, age, latitude, season and quality of the sample, etc.). Researchers have proposed this definition: the true definition of hypovitaminosis D corresponds, as closely as possible, to the concentration of 25 OH D3 below which, in healthy subjects, PTH increases significantly [7].

Sources of vitamin D

Food	Quantity	Vitamin D content (IU)
Cod liver oil	15 ml	1400
Fresh wild salmon	100 g	600-100
Sardines, herring, canned tuna	100 g	224-332
Farmed salmon	100 g	100-250
Dried Chiitake mushrooms	100 g	1600
Dried flapjacks	100 g	130
Margarines	15 ml	65-110
Egg yolk	1	40
Yoghurt	100 g	89
Hard cheese	100 g	44
Parmesan cheese	100 g	28

II. Hypovitaminosis D

11.1 Epidemiological data

11.1.1 Hypovitaminosis D throughout the world :

Hypovitaminosis D is a public health problem worldwide. Its prevalence varies from 30 to 80% [13]. In 2007, Holick found that around 1 billion people worldwide suffer from vitamin D deficiency [14]. Vitamin D deficiency is increasingly common in children and is often under-diagnosed [8].

A cohort study carried out in Saudi Arabia, in the sunny eastern region, revealed a high prevalence of hypovitaminosis D of 65% [14]. In 2002, in Tunisia, a study including 389 women aged between 20 and 60 showed a prevalence of 48% [15].

11.1.2 Hypovitaminosis D in the paediatric population :

An increase in vitamin D deficiency in children and adolescents has been noted over the last two decades [13]. In a Malaysian study involving 402 children aged between 7 and 12 years, 72.4% of children had vitamin D levels below 20 ng/ml. [16]. A national multicentre study carried out in France in 2014, including 326 healthy children aged between 6 and 10, showed that at least a third of the population studied was vitamin D deficient [17]. In Germany, [25 (OH) D] levels were <20 ng/ml in 60% of native children aged between 3 and 17 [18]. In an English study by Absoud et al involving 1,120 healthy children aged between 4 and 18, the prevalence of hypovitaminosis D was estimated at 40% [18]. In another study carried out by Cairncross et al, in 2012, in New Zealand, which included 1329 children aged between 2 and 5 years, the prevalence of hypovitaminosis D (vitamin D<75 nmol/ml) was 90% [19].

II.1.3 Frequency of hypovitaminosis D in asthmatic children :

Our study showed that 92% of the population studied had hypovitaminosis D, severe deficiency ([25 OH Vitamin D] <10ng/ml) was found in 18% of cases, moderate deficiency was reported in 45% of cases and insufficiency was found in 29% of patients. Normal status was found in only 8% of our population. In Tunisia, a case-control study (38 asthmatic children versus 30 controls), conducted by Tangour in 2014 [20], had revealed a high prevalence of hypovitaminosis D in both asthmatics and controls with respective rates of 66 and 60%. 25 (OH) D] was 17.5 and 20.75ng/ml in asthmatics and healthy children respectively. In an Italian study including 75 asthmatic children, normal vitamin D levels were present in only 9.4% of cases, which is consistent with our results [21].

II.2 Potential factors influencing vitamin D levels

II.2.1 Age

In our population, 68% of our patients were under 9 years of age and had a mean vitamin D concentration of 16.8ng/ml, slightly lower than the 9-11 age group, whose mean vitamin D concentration was 19.2ng/ml. This difference could be explained by lower sun exposure; 78% of our patients lived in enclosed homes, with less time spent outdoors due to a new lifestyle (children are increasingly drawn indoors by video games, television and mobile phones). Commonly consumed foods are naturally low in vitamin D [22]. In our country, few foods are fortified with vitamin D, and those that are are more expensive and not accessible to most people. Our study was consistent with the data in the literature. In an American study, the National Health and Nutrition Examination Survey (NHANES), the authors showed that the prevalence of serum 25(OH)D levels <75 nmol/ml was higher in children aged 6-11 years (73%) than in children aged 1-5 years (63%) [23]. Similarly, Nakanoa assessed the 25 OH D concentration of 290 healthy infants and young children aged between 0 and 48 months. Mean serum concentrations of 25 OH-D were significantly lower in the 0-5 month age group (19 ng/ml) than in the 5-15 month age group and in the 16-48 month age group (30 ng/ml). This difference could be explained by exclusive breastfeeding, which is low in vitamin D [24].

11.2.2 Gender

In our study, the difference between vitamin D and gender was not significant. However, the mean serum level in girls (15.5 ng/ml) was lower than that in boys (19 ng/ml). This low level in girls could be explained by the wearing of long-sleeved clothing, a limited outdoor lifestyle, protection by sun creams and the small size of the sample. On the other hand, the US National Health and Nutrition Examination Survey (2001-2006) assessed [25 (OH) D] in children aged between 1 and 11 years, according to gender, and showed that the prevalence of vitamin D deficiency was 71% in girls compared with 67% in boys, although this difference was not statistically significant [23].

11.2.3 Phototype

Some studies have shown that vitamin D levels in fair skin are increased after 10 minutes' exposure, as opposed to dark skin, where less vitamin D is synthesised [25]. In our study, this was not the case as most of our patients had dark skin. The NHANES study [23] showed that serum 25 (OH) D levels <75 nmol/l were higher in black children (92%) than in white children (59%).

Meanwhile, an Italian study [21] of 427 healthy adolescents aged 1021 revealed that black adolescents had a higher prevalence of severe vit D deficiency than white subjects (35.3% vs 7.8%; p = 0.002).

II.2.4 Body mass index

Our study showed no significant association between serum vitamin D levels and BMI. 25 (OH) D] was almost the same in asthmatics with a normal BMI (17.9ng/ml) and those who were overweight (18.1ng/ml). This could be explained by the small sample size. On the other hand, this rate collapsed in obese patients (9.7ng/ml). This is consistent with data in the literature, given that obesity or overweight affects the bioavailability of vitamin D, which is thought to be sequestered in fat mass compartments [5]. An Italian study of 427 healthy adolescents aged 10-21 years showed that [25 (OH) D] was inversely proportional to BMI (p= 0.007) [23,27]. Direct measurement of body fat, alongside body mass index, could provide a more sensitive relationship between vitamin D concentration and obesity in children [16].

II.2.5 Housing zone and conditions

Our study showed no association between [25 OH D] and area of residence. 25 OH D] in patients living in urban areas was lower than in patients living in rural areas (16.8 ng/ml versus 19.3 ng/ml). This may be related to the fact that patients living in rural areas spent more time outdoors. In addition, [25 OH D] levels in patients living in damp houses were lower (16.2 ng/ml) than in those living in sunny houses (17.9 ng/ml). This was reported in a study by Checkley et al in 2016 which showed that vitamin D levels were low in an urban compared to a rural setting in two equatorial populations [27].

II.2.6 Duration of exposure to the sun

We chose not to include this parameter, given the subjectivity of the responses from the parents of the patients included. A questionnaire containing targeted and objective responses concerning this parameter has not yet been validated in the literature. However, studies have shown a significant direct positive correlation between the duration of exposure to the sun and the increase in [25 (OH) D]. In New Delhi (India), a study of schoolgirls aged between 6 and 18 showed a significant correlation between [25 (OH) D], the duration of exposure to the sun (p=0.001) and the percentage of body surface exposed (p=0.004) [28]. In Qatar, a cross-sectional study of 650 healthy subjects aged under 16. [29] showed that 57.5% of vitamin D-deficient subjects had no exposure to the sun. However, exposure to the sun remains the main source of vitamin D in the body. It accounts for almost 90% of our needs. It is estimated that exposure to the sun, arms and legs, for 5 to 30 minutes, twice a week, between 10 and 15 H in spring, summer and autumn, significantly increases 25(OH) levels [30].

II.2.7 Socio-economic level

Our study showed no association between serum vitamin D levels and socio-economic status. Paradoxically, [25 (OH) D] levels in children from a good socio-economic background were lower than those from an average or poor socio-economic background (14.2 ng/l versus 19 ng/ml). Similar results were demonstrated by a randomised study of schoolgirls in Delhi [28], aged 6-18, from different socio-economic backgrounds. Vitamin D deficiency was frequent in both groups, 89.6% in girls from low socio-economic backgrounds versus 91.9% in those from high socio-economic backgrounds. This could be explained by the fact that children from 'rich' families spent less time outdoors and were therefore less exposed to UV rays, but also by the lack of knowledge about the benefits of vitamin D.

11.2.8 Dietary intake of vitamin D

The exogenous intake of vitamin D could not be quantified in our study because most of the participants had an average or low socio-economic level (80%), which does not encourage them to consume products fortified with this vitamin, as these products are expensive on the market. What's more, the foods that are richest in vitamin D are products that are not commonly found in children's daily diets. A randomised study of 290 healthy schoolgirls aged between 6 and 17 showed a significant relationship between [25 OHD] and dietary intake of this vitamin [31].

11.2.9 Physical activity and vitamin D

Low levels of physical activity are currently recognised as a risk factor for vitamin D deficiency. In a cross-sectional study carried out in Saudi Arabia involving 503 pre-school children, 63% of the children were vitamin D deficient, and outdoor physical inactivity was significantly correlated with vitamin D deficiency ($p<0.001$)[32].

11.2.10 Geographical location

The amount of ultraviolet light reaching the earth's surface depends on where we are on the globe (altitude), the time of day and pollution [33]. Vitamin D levels are significantly correlated with altitude: the closer we are to the equator (the lower the altitude), the higher the vitamin D level [34].

II.2.11 Pollution

Some studies have shown that pollution reduces photosynthesis of vitamin D. Pollution absorbs ultraviolet rays which become unavailable for skin synthesis of vitamin D [33].

III. Interaction between asthma and vitamin D

The role of vitamin D in the primary prevention of asthma is an area of active investigation and stems from preclinical studies, mainly supported by the involvement of vitamin D in lung growth and the development of the immune system [35-36]. A reduced risk of asthma in mothers with 25 OHD levels in maternal or cord blood was demonstrated in a meta-analysis of 15 prospective studies involving 12758 participants and 1795 cases of asthma [36]. In a French study (EDEN study) [37] conducted by Baiz N et al in 2013, including 239 cord blood samples, 25 (OH) D levels were analysed and the children were followed up until the age of 5 using internationally validated questionnaires. This study investigated the association between the value of 25 (OH) D and the occurrence of asthma, allergic rhinitis or atopic dermatitis from birth to 5 years of age; the mean level of 25 (OH) D was 17.8 ng/ml. An inverse association was observed between cord blood 25 (OH) D levels and the risk of transient wheezing and atopic dermatitis. There was no association with asthma or allergic rhinitis at 5 years. Several reviews have shown the protective role of vitamin D in the prevention of asthma and other allergic manifestations, without being able to establish a causal relationship [39,40]. However, the protective role of this vitamin is controversial, as demonstrated by the following studies. It has been shown that certain VDR polymorphisms predispose to asthmatic disease. In fact, genetic studies of asthma have identified several chromosomal sites that are linked to the disease, including chromosome 12 (region q13-23). As the VDR is encoded by the q12 region, an association between

VDR polymorphisms such as the FOKI variant of the VDR and a genetic susceptibility to atopy and asthma has been reported; vitamin D is thought to act on the TH1/TH2 balance; vitamin D deficiency promotes TH2 imbalance, stimulation of TH17 cells and inhibition of Treg cells [40].

111.1Impact of vitamin D deficiency on asthma severity :

Apart from its role in the onset of asthma, vitamin D deficiency is thought to be associated with greater severity of asthmatic disease.

111.1.1Vitamin D deficiency and bronchial hyperreactivity :

The relationship between vitamin D deficiency and bronchial hyperresponsiveness has been studied by Chinellato et al. In a study including 45 children with mild to moderate asthma, vitamin D levels were significantly lower in patients with exercise-induced bronchoconstriction (assessed by spirometry) than in those without [33]. Bossé et al recently demonstrated that VDR is present in bronchial smooth muscle cells and thus acts directly in the bronchi [32]. Damera et al hypothesised that vitamin D would reduce the proliferation of bronchial smooth muscle and thus inhibit bronchial remodelling, via calcitriol which, by binding to the VDR, inhibits the production of thrombin and PDGF (Platelet Derived Growth Factor) via molecular mechanisms currently being identified: phosphorylation of a retinoblastic protein and activation of Checkpoint kinase [33].

III.1.2 Effect of vitamin D deficiency on respiratory function :

Vitamin D deficiency is thought to be responsible for impaired respiratory function. Indeed, Black et al have demonstrated the existence of a positive correlation between vitamin D levels and lung volumes in healthy subjects [34].

In a study carried out by Black et al in 2005, which included 14901 healthy individuals, it was shown that FEV1 and FVC were significantly lower in patients with a vitamin D level of less than 40 ng/ml, with a mean difference of 106 ml for FEV1 and 142 ml for FVC compared with people with a vitamin D level of more than 80 ng/litre. This deleterious effect of vitamin D deficiency on respiratory function has been reported in asthma in several other studies. Tolpannen et al reported similar results in a prospective study published in 2013 including 2259 children with a weak correlation between 25 (OH) D2 levels and FEV1 and FVC values [35]. Similarly, Chinellato et al, in an Italian study of asthmatic children, showed that there was a significant positive correlation between vitamin D levels and FVC (p=0.040) but not with FEV1 (p=0.157).

III.1.3 Vitamin D deficiency and therapeutic needs :

Two epidemiological studies by Brehm et al and Searing et al showed that vitamin D deficiency was associated with increased use of anti-inflammatory drugs in asthmatic children [35]. These studies therefore suggest that vitamin D deficiency increases the severity of asthma and increases therapeutic needs. Our results showed that mean vitamin D levels were lower in patients on ICs combined with a ß2LA than in children on ICs alone, although this association was not statistically significant.

III.2 Role of vitamin D deficiency in asthma control :

Chinelatto et al showed in a study including 75 Italian asthmatic children that vitamin D levels were positively correlated with the ACT (Asthma Control Test) and were higher in patients with controlled asthma than in patients with uncontrolled asthma [36]. In our study, the mean vitamin D concentration in patients with partially or uncontrolled asthma was lower than in patients with well-controlled asthma (13.12ng/ml versus 18.52 ng/ml; p=0.275), although the difference was not statistically significant.

III.2.1 Vitamin D and exacerbations :

Vitamin D could reduce the number of exacerbations in asthmatic children thanks to its anti-infectious role. In a Finnish study involving 284 children hospitalised for wheezing, vitamin D levels were inversely correlated with infection by respiratory syncitial virus (RSV) or rhinovirus [38]. In a study of two groups of asthmatic and non-asthmatic children conducted by Lee Jet al, it was also described that vit D potentiated the immune response against pneumococcus in atopic and asthmatic subjects [39]. Modulation of innate immunity suggests that vit D has anti-infectious properties. We now know that macrophages or monocytes exposed to an infectious agent such as the tuberculosis bacillus over-express Toll-likereceptor 2, VDR and 1-alpha hydroxylase.

III.2.2 Vitamin D and the risk of hospitalisation :

In a study carried out in Costa Rica, including 616 asthmatic children aged between 6 and 14 years, an increase in vit D levels was associated with a reduction in the number of hospital admissions for asthma attacks (p=0.03) and in the use of anti-inflammatory treatments during the previous year (p=0.01) [25]. This study also showed that vit D levels were inversely correlated with total IgE levels and the number of eosinophils in the blood [15]. These data are in agreement with the study published by Brehm et al which included 1024 children with mild to moderate persistent asthma in whom vitamin D insufficiency was associated with an increase in the number of hospitalisations and emergency room visits [29].

III. 2.3 Effect of vitamin D deficiency on response to corticosteroids :

It would appear that asthmatic children with insufficient or deficient levels of vitamin D responded less well to glucocorticoids than those with high levels of vitamin D. Further studies would be necessary to prove that this action of vitamin D on the pathways of corticoresistance would really translate into a clinical benefit for the patient.

IV. Vitamin D and future prospects :

IV. 1 Benefits of supplementation :

On the basis of these data, the value of vitamin D supplementation in preventing these exacerbations was studied. Majak et al were able to demonstrate in a double-blind study (vitamin D versus placebo) that vitamin D supplementation (500 IU of cholecalciferol) during the period between September and December in asthmatic children aged between 5 and 18 years led to a reduction in the number of exacerbations of infectious origin, even without an increase in blood vitamin D levels [41]. In a second randomised double-blind study carried out on Japanese schoolchildren to protect against influenza, vitamin D supplementation at a dose of 1200 IU every day for 4 months had a greater effect in the sub-group of asthmatic children and reduced the number of exacerbations by 93% compared with asthmatic children given a placebo. According to this study, vitamin D supplementation reduced the carriage of influenzae A virus (diagnosed by nasal swab) in these asthmatic children without altering the carriage of influenzae B virus [42]. A critical evaluation of the clinical benefits of vitamin D supplementation in asthma, as in dysimmune diseases, needs to be undertaken. The majority of studies to date have been epidemiological and observational, generating hypotheses but not proving causality. It is particularly difficult to cancel out the biases associated with the diseases themselves and with vitamin D levels, such as physical activity, milk consumption and body mass index.

Large-scale, multi-centre, randomised studies are therefore needed to determine precisely the effects of different doses of vitamin D on asthma genesis, severity and control.

IV. 2 Recommendations :

In Tunisia, vitamin D supplementation is currently only recommended for children from birth to 18 months of age. Some practitioners supplement certain patients with chronic pathologies that interfere with phospho-calcium metabolism.

Vitamin D testing and supplementation for asthmatic children are not part of our daily practice.

While it is not useful to carry out systematic tests, it is logical to recommend :

- Reasonable exposure to natural light in the form of outdoor activities,
- Regular consumption (within recommended limits) of oily fish, eggs, fortified dairy products, fortified vegetable oils and fortified cereals,
- Supplementation in the event of pathology linked to a deficiency, and for infants, the elderly and pregnant women,
- Subjects with little exposure to the sun or who are unable to ensure

Correct intakes [43].

Conclusions

In recent decades, there has been a growing body of literature on the subject of vitamin D, illustrating both the pandemic nature of hypovitaminosis D and its much wider involvement in human physiology. It is true that vitamin D is the key hormone in bone metabolism and the maintenance of phosphocalcium homeostasis, but numerous studies and experiments have suggested several potential non-classical effects of this prohormone exerted via its VDR receptor (Vitamin D Receptor), which is expressed on virtually every cell in the body. Expression of this receptor confers on vitamin D a direct action on pro-inflammatory cells, notably dendritic cells, lymphocytes, monocytes and epithelial cells, explaining in particular the immunomodulatory properties of this pro-hormone. Vitamin D deficiency or insufficiency could therefore be associated with increased susceptibility to infections, particularly respiratory infections, and with the development of certain autoimmune or inflammatory diseases, including asthma.

Asthma is a major public health problem throughout the world: its prevalence is on the rise in several countries, and its morbidity and mortality, especially in the event of severe exacerbations, are to be feared.

Asthma is defined as chronic inflammation of the airways, the pathogenesis of which is complex and not clearly understood. Genetic and environmental factors are thought to be involved in this heterogeneous scourge. Among the environmental factors, the vitamin D status of asthmatic children is thought to play a crucial role in the severity, control and response to corticosteroids. Numerous studies have shown that vitamin D supplementation can improve asthma control and lung function.

References

1. Global Initiative for Asthma (GINA). Global strategy for asthma management and prevention. 2019. Available at URL: http://www.ginaasthma.org/.

2. Delmas MC, Guignon N, Leynaert B, Moisy M, Marguet C, Fuhrman C. Increasing prevalence of asthma in young children in France. Rev Mal Respir. 2017;34:525-34.

3. Lougheed MD, Lemiere C, Ducharme FM. Canadian Thoracic Society 2012 guideline update: Diagnosis and management of asthma in preschoolers, children and adults. Can Respir J. 2012;19:127-64.

4. Dutau G. Vitamin D, immunity, asthma and symptoms of atopy Médecine & enfance. 2013;33 (4):117-305.

5. Souberbeille JC. Classical and non-classical effects of vitamin D Correspondences en Métabolismes Hormones Diabètes et Nutrition.2011;5, 163-71

6. Mailhot G; White JH. Vitamin D and Immunity in Infants and Children. Nutriments. 2020;12 :1233-62.

7. Souberbielle JC, Prié D, Courbebaisse M. Update on the effects of vitamin D and assessment of vitamin D status. Revue Francophone des laboratoires 2009;414:31-9.

8. Holick MF. The vitamin D deficiency pandemic: approaches for diagnosis, treatment and prevention. Rev Endocr Metab Disord. 2017;18:153-65.

9. Bener A, Ehlayel MS, Bener HZ, Qutayba Hamid Q. The impact of Vitamin D deficiency in asthmatic and allergic children. J Family Community Med. 2014; 21(3):154-16.

10. Rolland Cachera MF. Childhood obesity: current definitions and recommendations for their use. Int J Pediatr Obes. 2011; 6: 325-31.

11. Holick MF, Binkley NC, Bischoff-Ferrari HA, Gordon CM, Hanley DA, Heaney RP et al. Evaluation, treatment, and prevention of vitamin D deficiency: an Endocrine Society clinical practice guideline. J Clin Endocrinol Metab. 2011;96(7):1911-30

12. Souberbielle J-C. Vitamin D: metabolism and evaluation of reserves. La Presse Médicale. 2013; 42(10):1343-50

13. Holick MF. Vitamin D deficiency in 2010: health benefits of vitamin D and sunlight: a D-bate. Nat Rev Endocrinol. 2011;7(2):73-5.

14. Elsammak M, Al-Wossaibi A, Al-Howeish A, Alsaeed J. High prevalence of vitamin D deficiency in the sunny Eastern region of Saudi Arabia: a hospital-based study. Eastern Mediterranean Health Journal. 2011;17(4):317-22.

15. Meddeb N, Sahli H, Chahed M, Abdelmoula J, Feki M, Salah H, et al. Vitamin D deficiency in Tunisia. Osteoporosis International. 2005; 16 (2):180-3.

16. Khor GL, Chee W SS, Shariff ZM, Poh KB, Arumugam M, Rahman G et al. High prevalence of vitamin D insufficiency and its association with BMI-for-age among primary school children in Kuala Lumpur, Malaysia. BMC Public Health. 2011;11:95.

17. Bener A, Al-Ali M, Hoffmann GF. Vitamin D deficiency in healthy children in a sunny country: associated factors. International Journal of Food Sciences and Nutrition. 2009;60(suppl 5):60-70.

18. Hintzpeter B, Scheidt-Nave C, Müller MJ, Schenk L, Mensink GB. Higher prevalence of vitamin D deficiency is associated with immigrant background among children and adolescents in Germany. J Nutr. 2008;138(8): 1482-90.

19. Tolppanen AM, Sayers A, Granell R, Fraser WD, Henderson J, Lawlor DA. Prospective association of 25-hydroxyvitamin D3 and D2 with childhood lung function, asthma, wheezing, and flexural dermatitis. Epidemiology. 2013;24:310-9.

20. Tangour E. Role of vitamin D deficiency in the severity and control of childhood asthma [Thesis]. Medicine: Tunis; 2014. 51p.

21. Vierucci F, Del Pistoia M, Fanos M, Gori M, Carlone G, Erba P et al. Vitamin D status and predictors of hypovitaminosis D in Italian children and adolescents: a cross-sectional study. European journal of pediatrics. 2013; 172 (12): 1607-17

22. lOM (Institute of Medicine). Dietary reference intakes for calcium and vitamin D. Committee to review dietary reference intakes for calcium and vitamin D. Washington: National Academies Press; 2011.

23. Mansbach JM, Ginde AA, Camargo CA. Serum 25-hydroxyvitamin D levels among US children aged 1 to 11 years: do children need more vitamin D? Pediatrics. 2009;124 (5): 1404-10.

24. Nakano S, Suzuki M, Minowa K, Hirai S, Takubo N, Sakamoto Y, et al. Current Vitamin D Status in Healthy Japanese Infants and Young Children. Journal of nutritional science and vitaminology. 2018;64(2):99-105.

25. Briot K, Audran M, Cortet B, Fardellone P, Marcelli C, Orcel P, et al. Vitamin D: effect on bone and extra-bone; recommendations for correct use. La Presse Médicale. 2009;38 (1):43-54.

26. Yahyaoui S, Jmal L, Sammoud S , Abdenebi M , Jmal A, Boukthir S. Vitamin D deficiency is associated with metabolic syndrome in Tunisian children with obesity. Tun Med. 2019; 97(12):1353-6.

27. Checkley W, MD P, Robinson CL, MPH MD, Baumann ML, Hanse NN et al. 25-hydroxy vitamin D levels are associated with childhood asthma in a population based study in Peru. Clin Exp Allergy. 2015;45(1): 273-82.

28. Puri S, Marwaha RK, Agarwal N, Tandon N, Agarwal R, Grewal K et al. Vitamin D status of apparently healthy schoolgirls from two different socioeconomic strata in Delhi: relation to nutrition and lifestyle. British Journal of Nutrition. 2008;99(4):876-82.

29. Bener A, Al-Ali M, Hoffmann GF. Vitamin D deficiency in healthy children in a sunny country: associated factors. International journal of food sciences and nutrition. 2009; 60(sup5):

30. Audran M, Briot K. Critical analysis of vitamin D deficiency. Revue du Rhumatisme 2010;77:139-43.

31. Marwaha RK, Tandon N, Agarwal N, Puri S, Agarwal R, Singh S, et al. Impact of two regimens of vitamin D supplementation on calcium-vitamin D-PTH axis of schoolgirls of Delhi. Indian Pediatrics. 2010;47(9):761-9.

32. Kensarah OA, Jazar AS, Azzeh FS. Hypovitaminosis D in Healthy Toddlers and Preschool Children from Western Saudi Arabia. Int J Vitam Nutr Res. 2015;85 (1- 2):50-60.

33. Holick MF. Environmental factors that influence the cutaneous production of vitamin D. Am J Clin Nutr. 1995;61 Suppl3:S638-S45.

34. Carnevale V, Modoni S, Pileri M, Di Giorgio A, Chiodini I, Minisola S, et al. Longitudinal evaluation of vitamin D status in healthy subjects from southern Italy: seasonal and gender differences. Osteoporos Int. 2000;12(12):1026-30

35. Zosky GR, Berry LJ, Elliot JG, James AL, Gorman S, Hart PH. Vitamin D deficiency causes deficits in lung function and alters lung structure. Am J Respir Crit Care Med. 2011;183:1336-43.

36. Pfeffer PE, Hawrylowicz CM. Vitamin D in Asthma: Mechanisms of Action and Considerations for Clinical Trials. Chest. 2018;153:1229-39

37. Baiez Baïz N, Dargent PM, Wark JD, Souberbeille JC. Cord serum 25-hydroxyvitaminD and risk of early childhood, transcient wheezing and atopic dermatitis. 20. Vitamin D Levels. J allergy Clin immunol.2014; 133:147.

38. Izabela Szymczak I and Pawliczak R. Can vitamin D help in achieving asthma control? Vitamin D" revisited": an updated insight Adv Respir Med. 2018; 86:1039.

39. Saadoon A, Ambalavanan N, Zinn K, Ashraf AP, MacEwen M, Nicola T.

Effect of Prenatal versus Postnatal Vitamin D Deficiency on Pulmonary Structure and Function in Mice. Am. J. Respir. Cell Mol Biol. 2017.56:383-392

40. Garland C, Garland F, Gorham E, Lipkin M, Newmark H, Mohr S et al. The role of vitamin D in cancer prevention. Am J Public Health 2006:96(2):25261.

41. Schoindre Y, Terrier B, Kahn J-E, Saadoun D, Souberbielle J-C, Benveniste O, et al. Vitamin D and autoimmunity. First part: fundamental aspects. La Revue de Médecine Interne. 2012;33(2):80-6.

42. Erkkola M, Kaila M, Nwaru BI, Kronberg-Kippilä C, Ahonen S, Nevalainen J et al. Maternal vitamin D intake during pregnancy is inversely associated with asthma and allergic rhinitis in 5-year-old children. Clin Exp Allergy. 2009;39:875-82.

43. Sharief S, Jariwala S, Kumar J, Muntner P, Melamed ML. Vitamin D levels and food and environmental allergies in the United States: results from the National Health and Nutrition Examination Survey 2005-2006 J Allergy Clin Immunol. 2011;127:1195-202.

44. Mailhot G; White J H. Vitamin D and Immunity in Infants and Children. Nutriments. 2020; 12, 1233-62.

Evaluation du contrôle de l'asthme à partir de 6 ans selon GINA 2019

Durant les 4 dernières semaines, l'enfant a t il eu :	Bien contrôlé	Partiellement contrôlé	Non controlé
• Symptômes d'asthme transitoires la journée <u>plus de 2 fois</u> par semaine ? OUI ❑ NON ❑ • Un réveil ou une toux nocturne liés à l'asthme? OUI ❑ NON ❑ • Besoin de BD <u>plus de 2 fois</u> par semaine? OUI ❑ NON ❑ • Une limitation d'activité à cause de son asthme ? OUI ❑ NON ❑			

Équivalence de doses de corticoïdes inhalés

	Adultes/Ados			Enfants		
	Faible	Modérée	Forte	Faible	Modérée	Forte
Beclometasone CFC	200-500	500-1000	>1000	100-200	250-500	500-1000
Beclometasone HFA	100-200	200-400	>400	50-100	100-200	>200
Budésonide DPI	200-400	400-800	>800	<200	200-400	>400
Budésonide neb				250-500	500-1000	>1000
Fluticasone DPI/HFA	100-250	250-500	>500	<100	100-200	200-400
Ciclosenide HFA	80-160	160-320	> 320			
Mometasone furoate DPI	110-220	220-440	>440			

Assessment based on asthma control

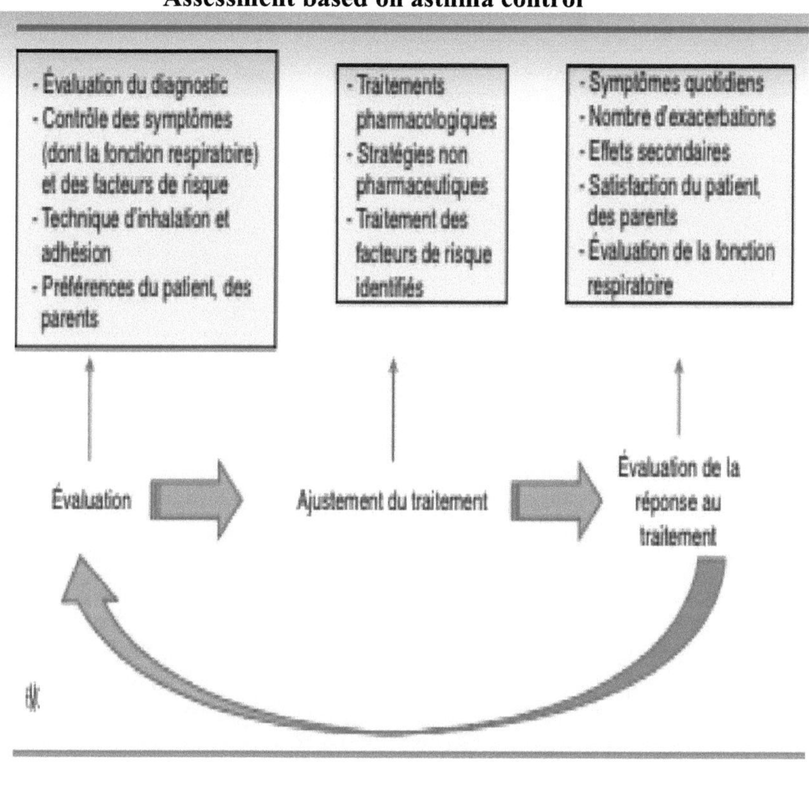

Staged asthma treatment strategy

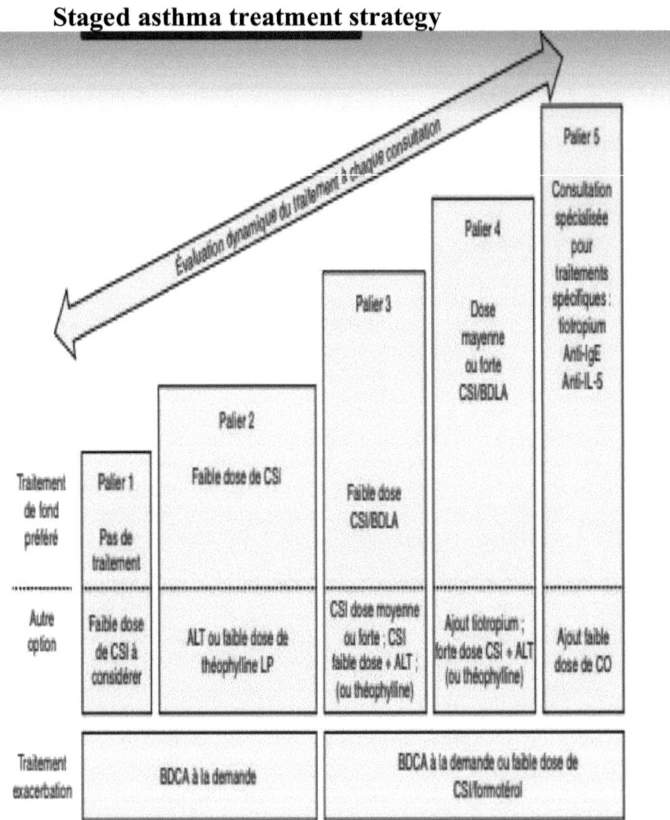

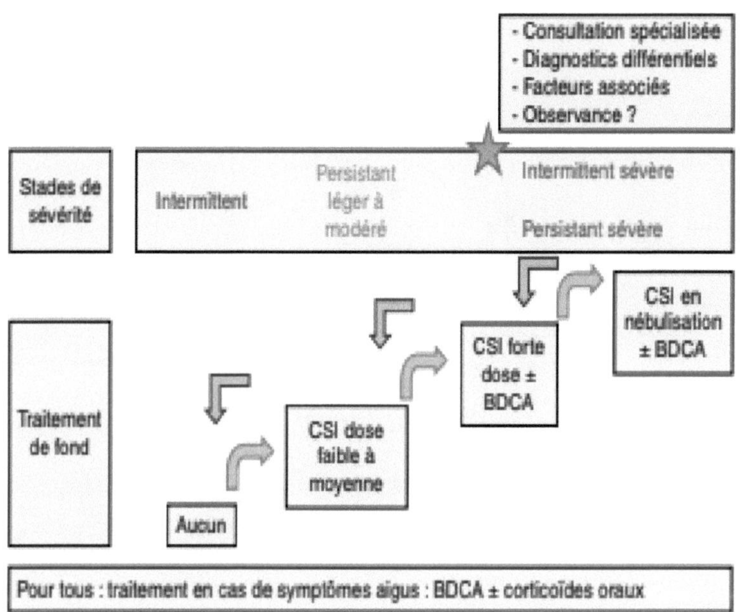
- Consultation spécialisée
- Diagnostics différentiels
- Facteurs associés
- Observance ?
Stades de sévérité
Intermittent
Persistant léger à modéré
Intermittent sévère
Persistant sévère
Traitement de fond
Aucun
CSI dose faible à moyenne
CSI forte dose ± BDCA
CSI en nébulisation ± BDCA
Pour tous : traitement en cas de symptômes aigus : BDCA ± corticoïdes oraux

Vitamin D metabolism

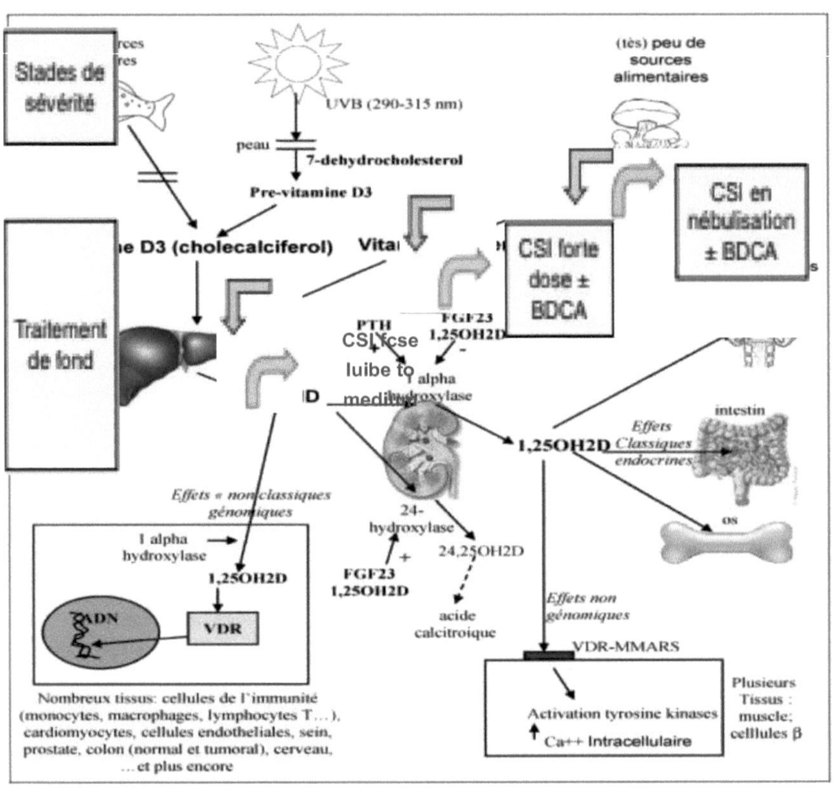

Definition of vitamin D status

Normes	Valeurs concentration	25-OH vitamine D
	ng/ml	nmol/l
Suffisantes	30-40	75-100
Insuffisantes	20-29	50-75
Déficit modéré	10 - 19	25- 50
Déficit sévère	< 10	<25
Taux recommandé	40-60	100-150
Intoxication	>150	>375

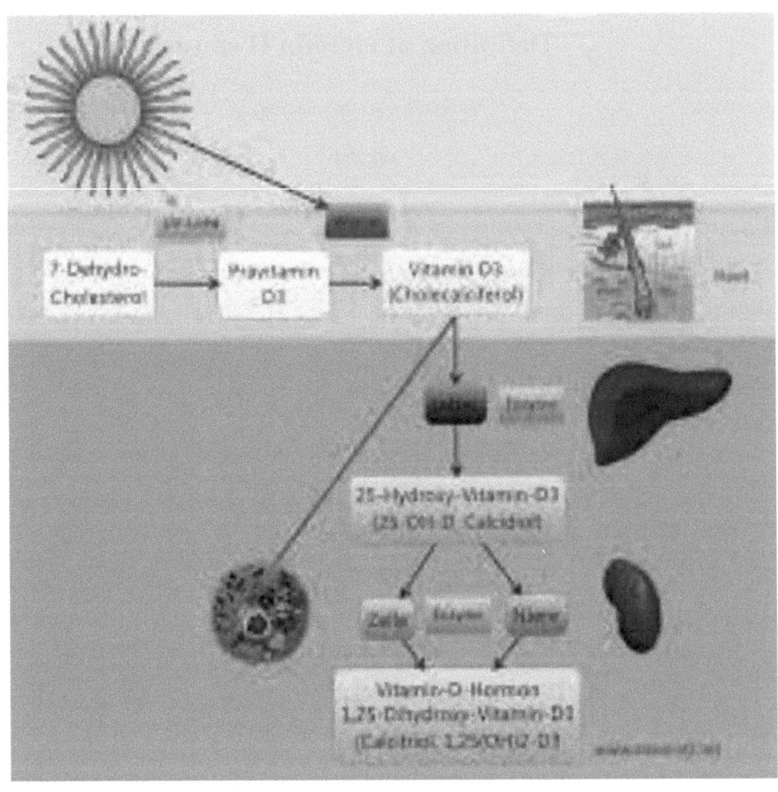
7-Dehydro-
Cholesterol
Prävitamin
D3
Vitamin D3
(Cholecalciferol)
25-Hydroxy-Vitamin-D3
Zelle
Niere
Vitamin-D-Hormon

Table of contents

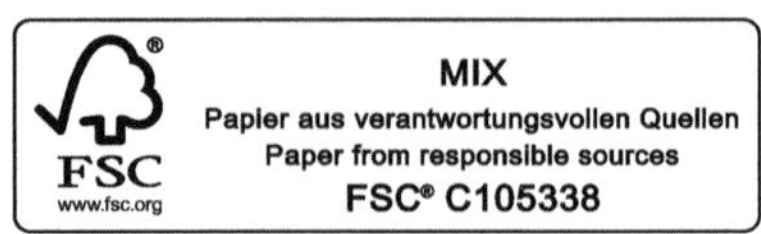

Printed by Books on Demand GmbH, Norderstedt / Germany